FIRST AID FOR NEPHROLOGY

A Comprehensive Pocket Guide: Key Concepts and Clinical Pearls

Dr Essam Abdelhakim

Copyright © 2024 Dr Essam Abdelhakim

All rights reserved

The characters and events portrayed in this book are fictitious. Any similarity to real persons, living or dead, is coincidental and not intended by the author.

No part of this book may be reproduced, or stored in a retrieval system, or transmitted in any form or by any means, electronic, mechanical, photocopying, recording, or otherwise, without express written permission of the publisher.

Cover design by: Art Painter
Library of Congress Control Number: 2018675309
Printed in the United States of America

CONTENTS

Title Page
Copyright
Disclosure
Introduction to Nephrology   1
Chapter 1: Renal Anatomy and Physiology   2
Chapter 2: Glomerular Diseases   7
Chapter 3: Glomerulonephritis   10
Chapter 4: Tubulointerstitial Diseases   13
Chapter 5: Acute Kidney Injury (AKI)   16
Chapter 6: Chronic Kidney Disease (CKD)   19
Chapter 7: Electrolyte and Acid-Base Disorders   21
Chapter 8: Hypertension and the Kidneys   24
Chapter 9: Nephrolithiasis (Kidney Stones)   27
Chapter 10: Dialysis and Renal Replacement Therapy   30
Chapter 11: Kidney Transplantation   33
Chapter 12: Genetic and Congenital Kidney Diseases   36
Chapter 13: Renal Pharmacology   39
Chapter 14: Q&A Section   43
Chapter 15: References   82
About The Author   83

DISCLOSURE

Disclosure

This book has been created with the assistance of ***Artificial Intelligence (AI) tools*** and thoroughly reviewed and edited by the author to ensure clarity, relevance, and educational value.

While every effort has been made to provide accurate and up-to-date information, this content is intended solely for educational and informational purposes.

The author is a medical professional; however, the information provided in this book *is not a substitute for professional medical advice, diagnosis, or treatment.*

Readers are strongly advised to consult licensed healthcare providers or specialists for any medical concerns or conditions.

By using this book, **you acknowledge and agree** that the author shall not be held responsible or liable for any loss, damage, or harm whether physical, emotional, financial, or otherwise that may occur *as a result of the use or misuse of the information presented herein.*

INTRODUCTION TO NEPHROLOGY

Welcome to the **Nephrology Essentials: A Comprehensive Guide for Medical Students and Residents**.

In this Book, we delve deeply into the most important topics within nephrology, providing a thorough understanding of the underlying pathophysiology, clinical presentation, diagnosis, and management of various renal conditions. The topics covered include:

1. **Chronic Kidney Disease (CKD)**
2. **Acute Kidney Injury (AKI)**
3. **Glomerular Diseases**
4. **Electrolyte and Acid-Base Disorders**
5. **Hypertension in Kidney Disease**
6. **Dialysis and Renal Replacement Therapy**
7. **Kidney Transplantation**
8. **Genetic and Congenital Kidney Diseases**
9. **Renal Pharmacology**

To further enhance your learning experience, the Book concludes with a **Q&A section** *that includes 50 different styles of questions.*

CHAPTER 1: RENAL ANATOMY AND PHYSIOLOGY

Renal Anatomy

Each kidney measures about 10-12 cm in length and weighs approximately 150 grams in adults.

The kidney is encased in a fibrous capsule and surrounded by perinephric fat, which protects it from trauma.

The renal hilum, located medially, is the entry and exit point for the renal artery, vein, lymphatics, nerves, and ureter.

Internally, the kidney is divided into two main regions: the cortex and the medulla.

The cortex, the outer region, contains the glomeruli, proximal and distal convoluted tubules.

The medulla, on the other hand, consists of renal pyramids, which are the sites of the loops of Henle and the collecting ducts.

The apex of each pyramid, known as the renal papilla, empties urine into minor calyces, which coalesce into major calyces, eventually forming the renal pelvis that leads into the ureter.

Nephron: The Functional Unit Of The Kidney

Each kidney contains approximately 1 million nephrons.
A nephron consists of the renal corpuscle and the renal tubule.

1. **Renal Corpuscle**: Comprising the glomerulus and Bowman's capsule, this is where blood filtration begins. The glomerulus is a network of capillaries with a selectively permeable membrane that filters

blood based on size and charge, allowing water and small solutes to pass while retaining large molecules like proteins and cells. Bowman's capsule encases the glomerulus and collects the filtrate.

2. **Renal Tubule**: The filtrate then passes through the renal tubule, which is divided into the proximal convoluted tubule (PCT), loop of Henle, distal convoluted tubule (DCT), and collecting duct. Each segment of the tubule has distinct functions:
    - **PCT**: Reabsorbs about 65-70% of the glomerular filtrate, including water, ions (sodium, potassium, chloride), glucose, amino acids, and bicarbonate.
    - **Loop of Henle**: Creates a hyperosmolar medullary interstitium via the countercurrent multiplication mechanism, essential for concentrating urine.
    - **DCT**: Involved in the fine-tuning of sodium, potassium, and calcium excretion under hormonal influence (e.g., aldosterone and parathyroid hormone).
    - **Collecting Duct**: Regulates water reabsorption under the control of antidiuretic hormone (ADH), determining the final concentration of urine.

Renal Blood Flow And Filtration

The kidneys receive about 20-25% of cardiac output, highlighting their critical role in maintaining homeostasis.

Renal blood flow begins at the renal artery, which branches into smaller arterioles leading to the glomerulus.

Blood is filtered in the glomerulus, with the remaining blood exiting via the efferent arteriole, which gives rise to the peritubular capillaries and vasa recta that supply the nephron and participate in reabsorption and secretion processes.

The filtration barrier of the glomerulus consists of three layers: the endothelial cells, the glomerular basement membrane, and the podocytes.

These layers work together to selectively filter blood, ensuring that essential proteins and cells remain in the circulation while waste products and excess substances are excreted.

Functions Of The Kidney

1. **Excretion of Metabolic Waste Products**: The kidneys filter blood to remove metabolic waste products, such as urea, creatinine, and uric acid, which are excreted in the urine.
2. **Regulation of Blood Pressure**: The kidneys regulate blood pressure through the renin-angiotensin-aldosterone system (RAAS) and by modulating fluid balance and systemic vascular resistance.
3. **Electrolyte Balance**: The kidneys maintain electrolyte homeostasis by adjusting the excretion or reabsorption of key ions such as sodium, potassium, calcium, magnesium, and phosphate.
4. **Acid-Base Balance**: The kidneys regulate the body's acid-base status by reabsorbing bicarbonate and

excreting hydrogen ions and ammonium. They are the long-term regulators of acid-base balance, complementing the respiratory system.

5. **Erythropoiesis**: The kidneys produce erythropoietin, a hormone that stimulates red blood cell production in response to hypoxia.
6. **Vitamin D Metabolism**: The kidneys convert inactive vitamin D into its active form, calcitriol, which is essential for calcium and phosphate metabolism.

Renal Physiology In Disease

Understanding renal physiology provides insight into how various diseases can affect kidney function.

For example, in chronic kidney disease (CKD), there is a progressive loss of nephron function, leading to impaired filtration, electrolyte imbalances, and anemia due to reduced erythropoietin production.

Acute kidney injury (AKI) involves a sudden decrease in kidney function, which can result from prerenal (e.g., hypovolemia), intrinsic (e.g., glomerulonephritis), or postrenal (e.g., obstruction) causes.

CHAPTER 2: GLOMERULAR DISEASES

Glomerular diseases encompass a broad range of conditions that affect the glomeruli, the filtering units of the kidney.

These diseases can be categorized into primary glomerular diseases, where the kidney is the primary organ affected, and secondary glomerular diseases, where systemic conditions impact the kidneys.

Primary Glomerular Diseases

1. **Minimal Change Disease (MCD)**: MCD is the most common cause of nephrotic syndrome in children. It is characterized by diffuse effacement of podocyte foot processes, which is typically only visible on electron microscopy. Patients present with proteinuria, hypoalbuminemia, hyperlipidemia, and edema. Treatment usually involves corticosteroids, which often lead to remission.

2. **Focal Segmental Glomerulosclerosis (FSGS)**: FSGS is a heterogeneous disease characterized by sclerosis (scarring) in parts of some glomeruli. It can be idiopathic or secondary to other conditions like obesity, HIV, or heroin use. Patients present with proteinuria, which may be nephrotic or non-nephrotic, and progression to chronic kidney disease is common. Treatment includes corticosteroids, immunosuppressants, and management of underlying conditions.

3. **Membranous Nephropathy**: This is a common cause of nephrotic syndrome in adults and is characterized by the thickening of the glomerular basement membrane due to immune complex deposition. Causes can be idiopathic or secondary to infections, malignancies, or autoimmune diseases. Patients often present with proteinuria, and treatment depends on the severity, ranging from conservative management to immunosuppressive therapy.

4. **IgA Nephropathy (Berger's Disease)**: The most common glomerulonephritis worldwide, IgA nephropathy is characterized by the deposition of IgA in the glomeruli. It typically presents with episodic hematuria, often following respiratory or gastrointestinal infections. The disease course is variable, ranging from benign hematuria to progressive renal failure. Management includes controlling hypertension, using ACE inhibitors or ARBs, and in some cases, immunosuppressive therapy.

Secondary Glomerular Diseases

1. **Diabetic Nephropathy**: A leading cause of chronic kidney disease and end-stage renal disease, diabetic nephropathy results from long-standing diabetes mellitus. It is characterized by hyperfiltration, glomerular hypertrophy, and the eventual development of glomerulosclerosis. Patients present with proteinuria, which progresses to nephrotic syndrome, and eventually, renal failure. Management includes strict glycemic control, blood pressure control, and the use of ACE inhibitors or ARBs.

2. **Lupus Nephritis**: A complication of systemic lupus erythematosus (SLE), lupus nephritis results from immune complex deposition in the glomeruli. It presents with a range of symptoms, from mild hematuria and proteinuria to severe nephrotic syndrome or rapidly progressive glomerulonephritis. The treatment is based on the severity and may include corticosteroids, immunosuppressants, and biological agents.

3. **Post-Infectious Glomerulonephritis**: Often following a streptococcal infection, post-infectious glomerulonephritis is characterized by immune complex deposition in the glomeruli, leading to inflammation. Patients typically present with hematuria, proteinuria, hypertension, and edema. Treatment is supportive, including managing hypertension and edema.

CHAPTER 3: GLOMERULONEPHRITIS

Glomerulonephritis refers to a group of diseases that cause inflammation of the glomeruli, leading to impaired kidney function.

It can be primary (affecting only the kidneys) or secondary (associated with systemic diseases).

Classification And Pathophysiology

Glomerulonephritis can be classified based on the underlying mechanism and the appearance of the glomeruli on biopsy:

- **Acute Glomerulonephritis**: Rapid onset of symptoms such as hematuria, proteinuria, hypertension, and edema. Post-infectious glomerulonephritis is a common cause.
- **Chronic Glomerulonephritis**: Slow progression of symptoms over months to years, leading to chronic kidney disease. It can result from unresolved acute glomerulonephritis or primary diseases like IgA nephropathy.
- **Rapidly Progressive Glomerulonephritis (RPGN)**: A severe form that leads to rapid loss of kidney function within weeks to months. RPGN is often associated with crescent formation on kidney biopsy and can be caused by diseases like Goodpasture syndrome and ANCA-associated vasculitis.

Clinical Presentation

The clinical presentation of glomerulonephritis varies depending on the severity and type of disease:

- **Hematuria**: Often the first sign, hematuria can be microscopic or macroscopic (visible to the naked eye).
- **Proteinuria**: A common finding, proteinuria can range from mild to nephrotic syndrome levels (>3.5 g/day).
- **Hypertension**: Often present due to salt and water retention.
- **Edema**: Particularly in the face and lower extremities, due to hypoalbuminemia and salt retention.
- **Renal Function Decline**: May manifest as increased serum creatinine and decreased GFR.

Diagnosis

Diagnosis of glomerulonephritis involves a combination of clinical evaluation, laboratory tests, and kidney biopsy:

- **Urinalysis**: Reveals hematuria, proteinuria, and often red blood cell casts.
- **Blood Tests**: Include serum creatinine, complement levels, and tests for specific antibodies (e.g., anti-streptolysin O, anti-GBM, ANCA).
- **Kidney Biopsy**: Provides definitive diagnosis by revealing the specific pattern of glomerular injury, such as immune complex deposition, crescent formation, or sclerosis.

Management

Treatment of glomerulonephritis depends on the underlying cause and severity:

- **Immunosuppressive Therapy**: Corticosteroids, cyclophosphamide, and other immunosuppressants are used in conditions like lupus nephritis, ANCA-associated vasculitis, and IgA nephropathy.
- **Plasmapheresis**: May be indicated in severe cases, such as Goodpasture syndrome or RPGN, to remove pathogenic antibodies.
- **Supportive Care**: Includes managing hypertension, proteinuria, and complications of chronic kidney disease. ACE inhibitors or ARBs are often used to reduce proteinuria and slow disease progression.

CHAPTER 4: TUBULOINTERSTITIAL DISEASES

Tubulointerstitial diseases affect the renal tubules and interstitium, rather than the glomeruli. These conditions can lead to chronic kidney disease and are often the result of infections, toxins, or systemic diseases.

Acute Tubulointerstitial Nephritis (Atin)

ATIN is characterized by inflammation of the renal interstitium and tubules, often triggered by drugs (e.g., NSAIDs, antibiotics), infections, or autoimmune diseases.

Patients may present with acute kidney injury, hematuria, pyuria, and proteinuria.

The hallmark finding on biopsy is interstitial edema with a mixed inflammatory infiltrate, often containing eosinophils.

Treatment typically involves discontinuing the offending agent and administering corticosteroids in severe cases.

Chronic Tubulointerstitial Nephritis (Ctin)

CTIN represents a chronic, progressive form of tubulointerstitial nephritis, often leading to chronic kidney disease.

Causes include prolonged exposure to nephrotoxins (e.g., NSAIDs, lithium), chronic infections, and systemic diseases like sarcoidosis and Sjögren's syndrome. Histologically, CTIN is characterized by interstitial fibrosis, tubular atrophy, and mononuclear cell infiltration.

Management focuses on treating the underlying cause and slowing disease progression, often through supportive care, avoiding further nephrotoxic exposure, and managing complications like hypertension and electrolyte imbalances.

Acute Pyelonephritis

Acute pyelonephritis is a bacterial infection of the renal parenchyma and renal pelvis, often resulting from ascending infection from the lower urinary tract.

Common pathogens include E. coli, Proteus, and Klebsiella species.

Patients typically present with fever, flank pain, dysuria, and urinary frequency. Urinalysis often reveals pyuria, bacteriuria, and sometimes white blood cell casts.

Treatment involves antibiotics tailored to the causative organism, and hospitalization may be required in severe cases.

Chronic Pyelonephritis

Chronic pyelonephritis is associated with recurrent urinary tract infections and can lead to scarring of the renal parenchyma and chronic kidney disease.

It is often seen in patients with urinary tract abnormalities such as vesicoureteral reflux or obstructive uropathy.

Symptoms may be subtle or absent, with patients presenting with hypertension or chronic kidney disease.

Diagnosis is based on imaging studies showing renal scarring and a history of recurrent infections.

Treatment involves managing urinary tract abnormalities and preventing further infections.

Analgesic Nephropathy

Analgesic nephropathy is a form of chronic tubulointerstitial nephritis caused by the long-term use of analgesics, particularly those containing phenacetin, aspirin, or acetaminophen.

The condition leads to papillary necrosis and chronic kidney disease.

Patients may present with non-specific symptoms like fatigue, hematuria, or signs of chronic kidney disease. Diagnosis is based on a history of analgesic use, imaging findings of small, scarred kidneys, and sometimes calcifications in the renal papillae.

Prevention is key, involving education on the risks of chronic analgesic use and managing pain with safer alternatives.

CHAPTER 5: ACUTE KIDNEY INJURY (AKI)

Acute kidney injury (AKI) is a sudden decrease in kidney function, leading to an accumulation of waste products in the blood, electrolyte imbalances, and fluid dysregulation.

AKI is classified based on the location of the insult: prerenal, intrinsic renal, or postrenal.

Prerenal Aki

Prerenal AKI is the most common form and is caused by decreased renal perfusion, often due to hypovolemia, heart failure, or sepsis.

The kidneys themselves are structurally normal, and if the underlying cause is addressed promptly, kidney function can return to normal.

Laboratory findings typically show elevated blood urea nitrogen (BUN) to creatinine ratio (>20:1) and low fractional excretion of sodium (FeNa <1%).

Intrinsic Aki

Intrinsic AKI is caused by direct damage to the kidneys, which can occur in the glomeruli, tubules, interstitium, or vasculature.

The most common cause of intrinsic AKI is acute tubular necrosis (ATN), which can result from prolonged ischemia or exposure to nephrotoxins.

Other causes include acute interstitial nephritis (AIN) and glomerulonephritis.

Laboratory findings vary depending on the cause but may include hematuria, proteinuria, and casts in the urine (e.g., muddy brown casts in ATN).

Postrenal Aki

Postrenal AKI is caused by obstruction of the urinary tract, leading to a backup of urine and increased pressure within the kidneys.

Common causes include kidney stones, tumors, and benign prostatic hyperplasia (BPH).

Diagnosis is often based on imaging studies showing dilated ureters or kidneys (hydronephrosis).

Treatment involves relieving the obstruction, which may require catheterization, surgery, or other interventions.

Diagnosis And Management

The diagnosis of AKI is based on an increase in serum creatinine or a decrease in urine output.

Management depends on the underlying cause:

- **Prerenal AKI**: Restore renal perfusion through fluid resuscitation or treating the underlying cause (e.g., improving cardiac output in heart failure).
- **Intrinsic AKI**: Remove the offending agent (e.g., nephrotoxin), manage underlying conditions (e.g., treat glomerulonephritis), and provide supportive care, including fluid and electrolyte management.
- **Postrenal AKI**: Relieve the obstruction, which may involve catheterization, stent placement, or surgery.

CHAPTER 6: CHRONIC KIDNEY DISEASE (CKD)

Chronic kidney disease (CKD) is a progressive loss of kidney function over months to years, often leading to end-stage renal disease (ESRD) requiring dialysis or transplantation.

CKD is defined by the presence of kidney damage or a glomerular filtration rate (GFR) <60 mL/min/1.73 m² for three months or more.

Stages Of Ckd

CKD is classified into five stages based on GFR:
- **Stage 1**: GFR ≥90 mL/min/1.73 m² with evidence of kidney damage (e.g., proteinuria, hematuria).
- **Stage 2**: GFR 60-89 mL/min/1.73 m² with evidence of kidney damage.
- **Stage 3**: GFR 30-59 mL/min/1.73 m².
- **Stage 4**: GFR 15-29 mL/min/1.73 m².
- **Stage 5**: GFR <15 mL/min/1.73 m², indicating ESRD.

Causes Of Ckd

The most common causes of CKD are diabetes mellitus, hypertension, and glomerulonephritis. Other causes include polycystic kidney disease, recurrent pyelonephritis, and prolonged exposure to nephrotoxins.

Clinical Manifestations

CKD can present with a wide range of symptoms, depending on the stage and underlying cause:

- **Early stages**: Patients may be asymptomatic or present with mild symptoms like fatigue, hypertension, and proteinuria.
- **Advanced stages**: Symptoms include uremia (e.g., nausea, vomiting, pruritus), fluid overload (e.g., edema, shortness of breath), electrolyte imbalances (e.g., hyperkalemia, metabolic acidosis), and anemia.

Management

Management of CKD focuses on slowing disease progression, managing complications, and preparing for renal replacement therapy in advanced stages:

- **Slowing Progression**: Tight control of blood pressure (target <130/80 mmHg), blood glucose (in diabetics), and using ACE inhibitors or ARBs to reduce proteinuria.
- **Managing Complications**: Treating anemia with erythropoiesis-stimulating agents, managing hyperkalemia with dietary restrictions and medications, treating metabolic acidosis with bicarbonate, and managing bone-mineral disorders with phosphate binders and vitamin D analogs.
- **Renal Replacement Therapy**: For patients with ESRD, options include hemodialysis, peritoneal dialysis, and kidney transplantation.

CHAPTER 7: ELECTROLYTE AND ACID-BASE DISORDERS

Electrolyte and acid-base disorders are common in nephrology and can have significant clinical implications.

The kidneys play a central role in maintaining electrolyte balance and acid-base homeostasis.

Sodium Disorders

1. **Hyponatremia**: Defined as a serum sodium concentration <135 mEq/L, hyponatremia can be caused by water retention (e.g., SIADH, heart failure), sodium loss (e.g., diuretics, vomiting), or a combination of both. Symptoms range from mild (e.g., headache, nausea) to severe (e.g., seizures, coma). Management depends on the underlying cause and the severity of symptoms, with options including fluid restriction, sodium replacement, and addressing the underlying condition.

2. **Hypernatremia**: Defined as a serum sodium concentration >145 mEq/L, hypernatremia is usually caused by water loss (e.g., dehydration, diabetes insipidus) or sodium gain (e.g., hypertonic saline). Symptoms include thirst, lethargy, and in severe cases, seizures or coma. Treatment involves careful rehydration with hypotonic fluids, addressing the underlying cause, and monitoring serum sodium levels to avoid rapid correction.

Potassium Disorders

1. **Hypokalemia**: Defined as a serum potassium concentration <3.5 mEq/L, hypokalemia can result from increased loss (e.g., diuretics, vomiting), intracellular shift (e.g., insulin, alkalosis), or decreased intake. Symptoms include muscle weakness, cramps, and arrhythmias. Management involves potassium replacement (oral or intravenous) and addressing the underlying cause.
2. **Hyperkalemia**: Defined as a serum potassium concentration >5.0 mEq/L, hyperkalemia is often caused by decreased renal excretion (e.g., CKD, medications like ACE inhibitors), increased intake, or cell lysis (e.g., rhabdomyolysis). Symptoms include muscle weakness, arrhythmias, and cardiac arrest. Treatment includes stabilizing the cardiac membrane with calcium, shifting potassium intracellularly (e.g., insulin and glucose), and removing excess potassium (e.g., diuretics, dialysis).

Acid-Base Disorders

1. **Metabolic Acidosis**: Characterized by a low blood pH and low bicarbonate level, metabolic acidosis can result from increased acid production (e.g., lactic acidosis, ketoacidosis), decreased acid excretion (e.g., renal failure), or bicarbonate loss (e.g., diarrhea). The anion gap is used to categorize metabolic acidosis into high anion gap (e.g., ketoacidosis) and normal anion gap (e.g., diarrhea). Treatment involves addressing the underlying cause and, in severe cases, bicarbonate therapy.
2. **Metabolic Alkalosis**: Characterized by a high blood pH and high bicarbonate level, metabolic alkalosis can result from vomiting, diuretic use,

or hyperaldosteronism. It is classified as chloride-responsive or chloride-resistant based on the response to saline infusion. Management involves treating the underlying cause and correcting electrolyte imbalances.

3. **Respiratory Acidosis**: Caused by hypoventilation, leading to increased CO_2 and a decrease in blood pH. Common causes include chronic obstructive pulmonary disease (COPD), sedative overdose, and neuromuscular disorders. Treatment focuses on improving ventilation and treating the underlying condition.

4. **Respiratory Alkalosis**: Caused by hyperventilation, leading to decreased CO_2 and an increase in blood pH. Common causes include anxiety, pain, hypoxemia, and sepsis. Treatment involves addressing the underlying cause and, in some cases, breathing into a paper bag to increase CO_2 levels.

CHAPTER 8: HYPERTENSION AND THE KIDNEYS

Hypertension and kidney disease are closely linked, with hypertension being both a cause and a consequence of kidney disease.

Pathophysiology

Hypertension can lead to kidney damage through various mechanisms, including glomerular hypertension, hyperfiltration, and ischemia.

Conversely, kidney disease can lead to hypertension through sodium retention, activation of the renin-angiotensin-aldosterone system (RAAS), and impaired nitric oxide production.

Primary Hypertension

Primary (essential) hypertension is the most common form of hypertension, with no identifiable cause.

However, it is often associated with genetic predisposition, obesity, and lifestyle factors.

Kidney involvement in primary hypertension can lead to nephrosclerosis, a condition characterized by thickening and hardening of the renal arteries, which can progress to chronic kidney disease.

Secondary Hypertension

Secondary hypertension is caused by an underlying condition,

many of which are related to the kidneys:
- **Renal Artery Stenosis**: Narrowing of the renal artery leads to decreased renal perfusion, triggering the RAAS and resulting in hypertension. It can be caused by atherosclerosis or fibromuscular dysplasia.
- **Chronic Kidney Disease**: As CKD progresses, the kidneys' ability to regulate blood pressure diminishes, often leading to hypertension.
- **Primary Aldosteronism**: Excess production of aldosterone by the adrenal glands leads to sodium retention and hypertension. This condition can be caused by adrenal adenomas or hyperplasia.

Diagnosis And Management

Diagnosing hypertension involves measuring blood pressure and identifying any underlying causes through history, physical examination, and laboratory tests.

Ambulatory blood pressure monitoring may be used to confirm the diagnosis.

Management of hypertension in patients with kidney disease involves lifestyle modifications (e.g., reducing salt intake, weight loss), pharmacologic therapy, and treating underlying causes.

The choice of antihypertensive medications often includes:
- **ACE Inhibitors/ARBs**: These are preferred in patients with CKD, as they reduce proteinuria and slow disease progression.
- **Calcium Channel Blockers**: Often used in combination with ACE inhibitors or ARBs to achieve blood pressure targets.
- **Diuretics**: Thiazide diuretics are effective in treating hypertension in patients with mild to moderate

CKD, while loop diuretics are used in advanced CKD.

CHAPTER 9: NEPHROLITHIASIS (KIDNEY STONES)

Types Of Kidney Stones

Kidney stones can be classified based on their composition:
- **Calcium Stones**: The most common type, usually composed of calcium oxalate or calcium phosphate. Risk factors include hypercalciuria, hyperoxaluria, and low citrate levels.
- **Uric Acid Stones**: Formed in acidic urine and often associated with hyperuricemia or gout.
- **Struvite Stones**: Composed of magnesium ammonium phosphate, these stones are associated with urinary tract infections caused by urease-producing bacteria.
- **Cystine Stones**: Rare and occur in patients with cystinuria, a genetic disorder affecting cystine reabsorption in the kidneys.

Pathophysiology

The formation of kidney stones involves supersaturation of the urine with stone-forming substances, leading to crystallization.

Factors that influence stone formation include urine pH, volume, and the presence of inhibitors like citrate.

Clinical Presentation

Patients with kidney stones typically present with acute, severe flank pain (renal colic) that radiates to the groin, hematuria, nausea, and vomiting.

Smaller stones may pass spontaneously, while larger stones can cause obstruction, leading to hydronephrosis and potential kidney damage.

Diagnosis

Diagnosis is based on clinical presentation and imaging studies. Non-contrast CT scan is the gold standard for detecting kidney stones, as it provides detailed information about the size, location, and composition of the stones.

Ultrasound and plain X-rays can also be used, particularly in pregnant patients or when avoiding radiation is necessary.

Management

The management of kidney stones depends on the size, location, and composition of the stones, as well as the severity of symptoms:

- **Conservative Management**: For small stones (<5 mm), conservative management includes hydration, pain control with NSAIDs or opioids, and medications to facilitate stone passage (e.g., alpha-blockers like tamsulosin).
- **Surgical Management**: Larger stones or those causing significant symptoms may require surgical intervention, such as extracorporeal shock wave lithotripsy (ESWL), ureteroscopy, or percutaneous nephrolithotomy.
- **Prevention**: Preventive measures include increasing fluid intake, dietary modifications (e.g., reducing oxalate and sodium intake, increasing citrate intake), and medications to correct underlying metabolic abnormalities (e.g., thiazide diuretics for hypercalciuria, allopurinol for hyperuricemia).

CHAPTER 10: DIALYSIS AND RENAL REPLACEMENT THERAPY

Dialysis and renal replacement therapy (RRT) are critical interventions for patients with end-stage renal disease (ESRD) or acute kidney injury (AKI) when the kidneys can no longer adequately filter waste products, electrolytes, and fluids from the blood.

Types Of Dialysis

There are two primary types of dialysis: hemodialysis and peritoneal dialysis, each with distinct indications, advantages, and limitations.

Hemodialysis

Hemodialysis involves circulating the patient's blood through a machine (dialyzer) that filters waste products and excess fluids before returning the cleansed blood to the body.

- **Access**: Vascular access is required, typically through an arteriovenous fistula (AVF), arteriovenous graft (AVG), or a central venous catheter (CVC). AVFs are preferred due to lower infection and thrombosis rates.
- **Procedure**: Hemodialysis is usually performed in a dialysis center three times per week, each session lasting about 4 hours. Home hemodialysis is also an option for some patients.
- **Advantages**: Provides efficient clearance of toxins and fluids, is well-suited for patients with acute conditions or those who cannot perform self-care.

- **Disadvantages**: Requires frequent visits to a dialysis center, vascular access complications, and may lead to hypotension and muscle cramps during or after treatment.

Peritoneal Dialysis

Peritoneal dialysis *uses the patient's peritoneum (the lining of the abdominal cavity) as a natural filter.*

A dialysis solution is infused into the abdominal cavity, where it absorbs waste and excess fluids before being drained.

- **Access**: A permanent catheter is placed into the peritoneal cavity.
- **Types**:
  - **Continuous Ambulatory Peritoneal Dialysis (CAPD)**: The patient manually exchanges dialysis fluid several times a day.
  - **Automated Peritoneal Dialysis (APD)**: A machine performs exchanges overnight while the patient sleeps.
- **Advantages**: Offers greater flexibility, allows for home treatment, and preserves residual renal function better than hemodialysis.
- **Disadvantages**: Higher risk of peritonitis, requires patient compliance, and is less effective for patients with large body sizes or severe metabolic imbalances.

Indications For Dialysis

Dialysis is initiated when a patient has ESRD or AKI with symptoms of uremia, such as fatigue, anorexia, nausea, fluid overload, hyperkalemia, acidosis, or pericarditis.

Indications are summarized by the mnemonic "AEIOU":

- **A**: Acidosis (severe, refractory metabolic acidosis)
- **E**: Electrolyte imbalance (severe hyperkalemia)
- **I**: Intoxications (certain drug overdoses)
- **O**: Overload of fluid (refractory to diuretics)
- **U**: Uremic symptoms (e.g., encephalopathy, pericarditis)

Continuous Renal Replacement Therapy (Crrt)

CRRT is a form of dialysis used primarily in critically ill patients with AKI.

It is performed continuously over 24 hours in an intensive care unit (ICU) setting, offering gentle fluid and solute removal, which is better tolerated by hemodynamically unstable patients.

Complications Of Dialysis

- **Infections**: Particularly with CVCs and peritoneal dialysis catheters.
- **Hypotension**: Common during hemodialysis, often due to rapid fluid removal.
- **Electrolyte Imbalances**: Including hypokalemia, hypocalcemia, and hyperphosphatemia.
- **Dialysis Disequilibrium Syndrome**: A rare but serious condition caused by rapid changes in blood urea levels during dialysis, leading to cerebral edema.

CHAPTER 11: KIDNEY TRANSPLANTATION

Indications And Contraindications

Indications: *The primary indication for kidney transplantation is ESRD from various causes, including diabetic nephropathy, glomerulonephritis, polycystic kidney disease, and hypertensive nephrosclerosis.*

Contraindications: *Absolute contraindications include active infection, uncontrolled malignancy, severe cardiovascular disease, or active substance abuse.*

Relative contraindications include obesity, advanced age, or noncompliance with medical therapy.

Donor Types

- **Living Donor Transplantation**: A kidney is donated by a living individual, usually a relative or close friend. Living donor kidneys generally have better outcomes due to shorter ischemia times and better health of the donor organ.
- **Deceased Donor Transplantation**: A kidney is obtained from a person who has died, usually from brain death or circulatory death. These transplants are more common but associated with longer waiting times and slightly lower success rates compared to living donors.

Immunosuppression

After transplantation, patients require lifelong immunosuppressive therapy to prevent organ rejection.

The typical regimen includes:

- **Induction Therapy**: Given at the time of transplantation to reduce the risk of early rejection, often using monoclonal or polyclonal antibodies (e.g., basiliximab, thymoglobulin).
- **Maintenance Therapy**: A combination of drugs including calcineurin inhibitors (e.g., tacrolimus, cyclosporine), antiproliferative agents (e.g., mycophenolate mofetil), and steroids (e.g., prednisone). The goal is to balance the prevention of rejection with minimizing drug toxicity and the risk of infection.

Complications Of Kidney Transplantation

- **Acute Rejection**: Can occur within the first few months post-transplant. Symptoms may include fever, oliguria, and graft tenderness, though it can also be asymptomatic and detected only by a rise in serum creatinine.
- **Chronic Rejection**: A slow, progressive loss of graft function over years, often leading to fibrosis and chronic allograft nephropathy.
- **Infections**: Due to immunosuppression, patients are at increased risk for bacterial, viral, and fungal infections. Prophylactic measures and close monitoring are crucial.
- **Post-transplant Lymphoproliferative Disorder (PTLD)**: A rare but serious complication associated with EBV infection and immunosuppression.
- **Cardiovascular Disease**: The leading cause of death in transplant recipients, requiring aggressive

management of risk factors like hypertension, dyslipidemia, and diabetes.

Long-Term Management

Long-term management includes regular monitoring of graft function (e.g., serum creatinine, urine output), immunosuppressive drug levels, and screening for complications such as infections, malignancies, and cardiovascular disease.

Patient education and adherence to medical therapy are crucial for long-term success.

CHAPTER 12: GENETIC AND CONGENITAL KIDNEY DISEASES

Polycystic Kidney Disease (Pkd)

Polycystic Kidney Disease (PKD) is one of the most common genetic kidney disorders, characterized by the growth of numerous cysts in the kidneys, which can lead to renal enlargement, hypertension, and progressive kidney failure.

- **Autosomal Dominant PKD (ADPKD):** The most common form, caused by mutations in the PKD1 or PKD2 genes. It typically presents in adulthood with symptoms like hypertension, hematuria, flank pain, and progressive renal insufficiency.
- **Autosomal Recessive PKD (ARPKD):** A rarer, more severe form that presents in infancy or early childhood, often leading to renal and hepatic fibrosis.

Alport Syndrome

Alport Syndrome *is a genetic disorder characterized by progressive kidney disease, hearing loss, and eye abnormalities.*

It is usually inherited in an X-linked manner due to mutations in the COL4A5 gene, which affects the production of type IV collagen, a crucial component of the glomerular basement membrane.

Fabry Disease

Fabry Disease *is a rare X-linked disorder caused by a deficiency of the enzyme alpha-galactosidase A, leading to the accumulation of globotriaosylceramide (Gb3) in various tissues, including the kidneys, heart, and nervous system.*

Renal involvement typically manifests as proteinuria, progressive CKD, and ESRD.

Congenital Anomalies Of The Kidney And Urinary Tract (Cakut)

Congenital Anomalies of the Kidney and Urinary Tract (CAKUT) *encompass a wide range of structural abnormalities that occur during fetal development, including renal agenesis, renal hypoplasia, and vesicoureteral reflux.*

CAKUT is a leading cause of CKD in children.

Cystinosis

Cystinosis *is a rare autosomal recessive disorder caused by mutations in the CTNS gene, leading to the accumulation of cystine in various organs, including the kidneys.*

The most severe form, nephropathic cystinosis, presents in infancy with Fanconi syndrome and progresses to ESRD by early adulthood.

Diagnosis And Management

Diagnosis of genetic and congenital kidney diseases often involves a combination of clinical evaluation, family history, genetic testing, and imaging studies. Management varies depending on the specific condition but may include:

- **Supportive Care**: Blood pressure control, management of proteinuria, and treatment of CKD

complications.
- **Enzyme Replacement Therapy**: For conditions like Fabry disease.
- **Renal Replacement Therapy**: Including dialysis and transplantation for patients with ESRD.

CHAPTER 13: RENAL PHARMACOLOGY

Diuretics

Diuretics are among the most commonly used drugs in nephrology, used to manage hypertension, fluid overload, and electrolyte imbalances.

- **Loop Diuretics**: (e.g., furosemide, bumetanide) inhibit the Na-K-2Cl symporter in the thick ascending limb of the loop of Henle, leading to potent diuresis. They are used in conditions like heart failure, nephrotic syndrome, and hypercalcemia.
- **Thiazide Diuretics**: (e.g., hydrochlorothiazide, chlorthalidone) inhibit the Na-Cl symporter in the distal convoluted tubule. They are primarily used for hypertension and can help reduce calcium excretion in patients with nephrolithiasis.
- **Potassium-Sparing Diuretics**: (e.g., spironolactone, eplerenone) antagonize the effects of aldosterone in the distal nephron, reducing potassium excretion. They are often used in conjunction with other diuretics to prevent hypokalemia.
- **Carbonic Anhydrase Inhibitors**: (e.g., acetazolamide) inhibit carbonic anhydrase in the proximal tubule, leading to increased excretion of bicarbonate, sodium, and water. They are used for conditions like metabolic alkalosis and glaucoma.

Renin-Angiotensin-Aldosterone System (Raas) Inhibitors

RAAS inhibitors play a crucial role in managing hypertension, proteinuria, and CKD progression.

- **ACE Inhibitors (ACEIs)**: (e.g., enalapril, lisinopril) block the conversion of angiotensin I to angiotensin II, reducing vasoconstriction and aldosterone secretion. They are first-line therapy for patients with diabetic nephropathy and other proteinuric kidney diseases.
- **Angiotensin II Receptor Blockers (ARBs)**: (e.g., losartan, valsartan) block the effects of angiotensin II at its receptor, offering similar benefits to ACEIs with a lower risk of cough and angioedema.
- **Aldosterone Antagonists**: (e.g., spironolactone, eplerenone) block the effects of aldosterone on the distal nephron, reducing sodium retention and potassium excretion.

Antihypertensives

Managing blood pressure is critical in patients with kidney disease to prevent progression to ESRD.

- **Calcium Channel Blockers**: (e.g., amlodipine, diltiazem) inhibit calcium influx into vascular smooth muscle cells, causing vasodilation. They are effective in lowering blood pressure and reducing proteinuria in patients with CKD.
- **Beta-Blockers**: (e.g., metoprolol, atenolol) reduce heart rate and cardiac output, lowering blood pressure. They are particularly useful in patients with concomitant cardiovascular disease.

- **Vasodilators**: (e.g., hydralazine, minoxidil) directly relax vascular smooth muscle, reducing peripheral resistance. They are often used in resistant hypertension.

Drugs And Kidney Disease

Kidney disease significantly alters drug pharmacokinetics, requiring careful dose adjustments and monitoring to avoid toxicity.

- **Drug Dosing in CKD**: Many drugs are eliminated by the kidneys, and in patients with CKD, their clearance is reduced. This necessitates dose adjustments to avoid accumulation and toxicity.
- **Nephrotoxic Drugs**: Certain drugs can cause or exacerbate kidney injury, including nonsteroidal anti-inflammatory drugs (NSAIDs), aminoglycosides, and contrast agents. Avoidance or careful monitoring is required in patients with kidney disease.
- **Immunosuppressive Drugs**: Used in transplantation and glomerulonephritis, these drugs require careful monitoring to balance efficacy with the risk of infection and other side effects.

CHAPTER 14: Q&A SECTION

1. **Which of the following is a common cause of nephrotic syndrome in adults?**

a) Minimal change disease
b) Focal segmental glomerulosclerosis (FSGS)
c) Membranous nephropathy
d) Diabetic nephropathy
e) All of the above
Answer: e) All of the above
Explanation: All listed conditions can cause nephrotic syndrome in adults, with diabetic nephropathy being the most common in the general population.

2. **Which diuretic is most likely to cause hyperkalemia?**

a) Furosemide
b) Hydrochlorothiazide
c) Spironolactone
d) Acetazolamide
Answer: c) Spironolactone
Explanation: Spironolactone is a potassium-sparing diuretic, which can increase serum potassium levels.

3. **Which of the following is the preferred treatment for Goodpasture syndrome?**

a) Antibiotics
b) Plasmapheresis
c) ACE inhibitors
d) Calcium channel blockers
Answer: b) Plasmapheresis
Explanation: Plasmapheresis is used to remove

circulating anti-GBM antibodies in Goodpasture syndrome.

4. Which genetic disorder is associated with renal cysts and an increased risk of aneurysms?

a) Alport syndrome
b) Fabry disease
c) Polycystic kidney disease
d) Cystinosis

Answer: c) Polycystic kidney disease

Explanation: Polycystic kidney disease (PKD) is associated with renal cysts and an increased risk of intracranial aneurysms.

5. Which of the following drugs requires dose adjustment in CKD?

a) Amlodipine
b) Metoprolol
c) Enoxaparin
d) Prednisone

Answer: c) Enoxaparin

Explanation: Enoxaparin, a low molecular weight heparin, is primarily excreted by the kidneys and requires dose adjustment in CKD to prevent bleeding complications.

6.*Match the condition with the appropriate treatment*:

1. **Minimal change disease**
2. **Diabetic nephropathy**
3. **Hypertension in CKD**
4. **Hyperkalemia**
5. **Membranous nephropathy**

A. ACE inhibitors
B. Immunosuppressive therapy
C. Calcium channel blockers

D. Corticosteroids
E. Potassium-binding resins

Answers:
1. D. Corticosteroids
2. A. ACE inhibitors
3. C. Calcium channel blockers
4. E. Potassium-binding resins
5. B. Immunosuppressive therapy

Explanation:
- **Minimal change disease** typically responds well to corticosteroids.
- **Diabetic nephropathy** is managed with ACE inhibitors to reduce proteinuria and slow disease progression.
- **Hypertension in CKD** often requires calcium channel blockers, among other agents.
- **Hyperkalemia** can be treated with potassium-binding resins.
- **Membranous nephropathy** may require immunosuppressive therapy depending on the severity of proteinuria and response to conservative management.

7. Explain the pathophysiology of nephrotic syndrome.
Answer: Nephrotic syndrome is characterized by increased glomerular permeability to proteins, leading to massive proteinuria, hypoalbuminemia, and edema. The loss of protein, particularly albumin, reduces plasma oncotic pressure, causing fluid to shift from the intravascular to the interstitial space, resulting in edema.

8. What are the key features of acute kidney injury (AKI)?
Answer: AKI is characterized by a sudden decline in kidney function, leading to an accumulation of waste products (e.g., urea, creatinine), disturbances in fluid and electrolyte balance, and acid-base abnormalities. Common causes include prerenal (e.g., hypovolemia), intrinsic (e.g., acute tubular necrosis), and postrenal (e.g., obstruction) factors.

9. Describe the mechanism of action of loop diuretics.
Answer: Loop diuretics inhibit the Na-K-2Cl symporter in the thick ascending limb of the loop of Henle, leading to increased excretion of sodium, potassium, chloride, and water. This reduces fluid overload and decreases blood pressure.

10. What is the significance of proteinuria in chronic kidney disease?
Answer: Proteinuria is a marker of glomerular damage and a risk factor for progression to ESRD. It contributes to kidney damage by promoting inflammation and fibrosis. Reducing proteinuria is a key target in the management of CKD.

11. How does peritoneal dialysis differ from hemodialysis?
Answer: Peritoneal dialysis uses the patient's peritoneal membrane as a filter to remove waste and excess fluid, while hemodialysis involves circulating blood through a machine (dialyzer) outside the body. Peritoneal dialysis offers greater flexibility and is typically performed at home, while hemodialysis is often done in a clinic setting.

12. Which of the following is a common feature of nephrotic syndrome?

a) Hematuria
b) Hypoalbuminemia
c) Hyperkalemia
d) Azotemia
Answer: b) Hypoalbuminemia
Explanation: Nephrotic syndrome is characterized by massive proteinuria, which leads to hypoalbuminemia and subsequent edema.

13. What is the most common cause of end-stage renal disease (ESRD) in the United States?
a) Hypertension
b) Glomerulonephritis
c) Diabetes mellitus
d) Polycystic kidney disease
Answer: c) Diabetes mellitus
Explanation: Diabetes mellitus is the leading cause of ESRD, contributing to diabetic nephropathy.

14. Which diuretic works by inhibiting the Na-K-2Cl symporter in the thick ascending limb of the loop of Henle?
a) Thiazide diuretics
b) Loop diuretics
c) Potassium-sparing diuretics
d) Carbonic anhydrase inhibitors
Answer: b) Loop diuretics
Explanation: Loop diuretics like furosemide inhibit the Na-K-2Cl symporter, leading to significant diuresis.

15. Match the following kidney diseases with their primary histological feature:
1. Membranous nephropathy
2. Focal segmental glomerulosclerosis (FSGS)

3. Minimal change disease
4. IgA nephropathy
5. Diabetic nephropathy

A. Mesangial IgA deposition
B. Podocyte effacement
C. Thickened glomerular basement membrane with immune deposits
D. Kimmelstiel-Wilson nodules
E. Segmental glomerular sclerosis

Answers:
1. C
2. E
3. B
4. A
5. D

Explanation:
- Membranous nephropathy is characterized by a thickened glomerular basement membrane due to immune deposits.
- FSGS involves segmental glomerular sclerosis.
- Minimal change disease shows podocyte effacement under electron microscopy.
- IgA nephropathy is marked by mesangial IgA deposition.
- Diabetic nephropathy is associated with Kimmelstiel-Wilson nodules.

16. True or False: Autosomal recessive polycystic kidney

disease (ARPKD) typically presents in adulthood.
Answer: False
Explanation: ARPKD usually presents in infancy or early childhood, often leading to significant renal and hepatic involvement.

17. True or False: Hemodialysis is more commonly associated with infections than peritoneal dialysis.
Answer: False
Explanation: Peritoneal dialysis is more commonly associated with infections, specifically peritonitis, compared to hemodialysis.

18. What is the primary mechanism of action of ACE inhibitors in the treatment of chronic kidney disease?
Answer: ACE inhibitors block the conversion of angiotensin I to angiotensin II, leading to vasodilation, reduced blood pressure, and decreased glomerular pressure, which helps to reduce proteinuria and slow the progression of chronic kidney disease.

19. Explain the significance of proteinuria in nephrotic syndrome.
Answer: Proteinuria in nephrotic syndrome is a result of increased glomerular permeability. It leads to hypoalbuminemia, which decreases oncotic pressure and causes edema. Proteinuria also signifies glomerular damage and is a key marker of disease severity.

20. A 45-year-old man with a history of hypertension presents with sudden onset of severe flank pain and hematuria. His blood pressure is 170/100 mmHg. What is the most likely diagnosis?
Answer: Renal artery thrombosis or renal stone.

Explanation: The sudden onset of severe flank pain and hematuria in the context of hypertension raises suspicion for renal artery thrombosis or a renal stone. Imaging would be necessary to differentiate between the two.

21. A 30-year-old woman with type 1 diabetes presents with worsening edema and proteinuria of 4 g/day. What is the next step in her management?
Answer: Intensification of blood pressure control, preferably with an ACE inhibitor or ARB, and tighter glycemic control.
Explanation: The patient likely has diabetic nephropathy. ACE inhibitors or ARBs are essential for reducing proteinuria and slowing the progression of nephropathy.

22. The most common cause of glomerulonephritis worldwide is _____.
Answer: IgA nephropathy
Explanation: IgA nephropathy is the most common cause of glomerulonephritis globally.

23. _____ is the most commonly used access type for long-term hemodialysis.
Answer: Arteriovenous fistula (AVF)
Explanation: AVF is preferred for long-term hemodialysis due to lower rates of infection and thrombosis compared to other access types.

24. Calculate the estimated glomerular filtration rate (eGFR) for a 65-year-old male patient with a serum creatinine of 2.0 mg/dL using the Cockcroft-Gault formula. The patient weighs 70 kg.
Answer: eGFR = (140−age)×weight (kg)/ (serum creatinine×72)

= 36.5

Explanation: The Cockcroft-Gault formula is used to estimate the eGFR, which helps assess kidney function.

.

25. Place the following steps of peritoneal dialysis in the correct sequence:
A. Infusion of dialysis solution
B. Drainage of spent dialysis solution
C. Equilibration period
D. Connection to the dialysis machine

Answer:
1. D. Connection to the dialysis machine
2. A. Infusion of dialysis solution
3. C. Equilibration period
4. B. Drainage of spent dialysis solution

Explanation: These are the typical steps in the process of peritoneal dialysis.

26. Compare and contrast the pathophysiology of acute tubular necrosis (ATN) and acute interstitial nephritis (AIN).

Answer:
- **ATN**: Caused by ischemia or nephrotoxins leading to necrosis of tubular epithelial cells. Common in sepsis and hypotension.
- **AIN**: Caused by an immune-mediated reaction, often due to drugs like NSAIDs or antibiotics, leading to interstitial inflammation and tubular dysfunction.

Explanation: Both conditions result in AKI but have distinct etiologies and histopathological features.

27. **A 60-year-old man with chronic kidney disease stage 4 presents with a new onset of hyperkalemia (K+ = 6.5 mEq/L). How would you manage this patient?**

Answer: Management includes stopping any potassium-sparing medications, administering calcium gluconate to stabilize the myocardium, insulin with glucose to drive potassium intracellularly, and considering dialysis if the hyperkalemia is refractory.

Explanation: Hyperkalemia in CKD is a medical emergency, requiring prompt intervention to prevent arrhythmias.

28. **Explain how the renin-angiotensin-aldosterone system (RAAS) contributes to the progression of chronic kidney disease.**

Answer: The RAAS promotes vasoconstriction and sodium retention, leading to increased glomerular pressure, proteinuria, and glomerulosclerosis, which contribute to CKD progression.

Explanation: RAAS inhibitors are used in CKD to reduce proteinuria and slow disease progression.

29. **What is the prognosis of autosomal dominant polycystic kidney disease (ADPKD)?**

Answer: ADPKD often leads to ESRD by the age of 60 in many patients, necessitating dialysis or transplantation. However, the rate of progression can vary based on genetic mutations and environmental factors.

Explanation: Understanding the natural history of ADPKD helps in managing patient expectations and planning treatment.

30. **What is the effect of reduced renal function on the metabolism of drugs like digoxin?**

Answer: Reduced renal function decreases the clearance of digoxin, leading to an increased risk of toxicity. Dosage adjustments are required in CKD.
Explanation: Knowledge of pharmacokinetics is crucial in managing drug therapy in patients with renal impairment.

31. A 25-year-old woman presents with hematuria and flank pain. Urinalysis shows red blood cell casts. What is the most likely diagnosis?
Answer: Glomerulonephritis
Explanation: Red blood cell casts are indicative of glomerulonephritis, which often presents with hematuria and flank pain.

32. Describe the pathophysiology of hypertensive nephrosclerosis.
Answer: Chronic hypertension leads to arteriolar sclerosis and glomerular ischemia, resulting in glomerulosclerosis and interstitial fibrosis, ultimately causing CKD.
Explanation: Understanding the link between hypertension and kidney damage is key to preventing progression to ESRD.

33. What are the main indications for starting dialysis in a patient with CKD?
Answer: Indications include refractory hyperkalemia, uremic symptoms (e.g., pericarditis, encephalopathy), severe acidosis, and fluid overload unresponsive to diuretics.
Explanation: Early recognition of dialysis indications is critical in managing advanced CKD.

34. Interpret the following lab results in a patient with CKD: BUN 60 mg/dL, Creatinine 4.0 mg/dL, K+ 6.0 mEq/L.

Answer: The lab results indicate significant renal impairment with azotemia and hyperkalemia, likely requiring intervention such as dialysis.
Explanation: Interpreting lab values in the context of CKD helps guide treatment decisions.

35. Discuss the ethical considerations in offering a kidney transplant to an elderly patient with multiple comorbidities.

Answer: Ethical considerations include balancing the benefits of prolonged life and improved quality of life against the risks of surgery, immunosuppression, and the potential for complications due to comorbidities.
Explanation: Ethical decision-making in nephrology often involves complex considerations, particularly in resource allocation and patient selection for transplantation.

36. Correlate the presence of proteinuria with the prognosis of chronic kidney disease.

Answer: The degree of proteinuria correlates with the risk of progression to ESRD. Higher levels of proteinuria are associated with a worse prognosis and a faster decline in renal function.
Explanation: Monitoring proteinuria is essential in assessing the severity of CKD and guiding treatment.

37. Explain the mechanism by which ACE inhibitors reduce proteinuria in patients with diabetic nephropathy.

Answer: ACE inhibitors reduce angiotensin II-mediated efferent arteriolar constriction, thereby reducing glomerular hypertension and protein filtration, leading to decreased proteinuria.
Explanation: The renoprotective effects of ACE inhibitors are vital in managing diabetic nephropathy.

38. Describe the steps in initiating a peritoneal dialysis regimen in a patient with ESRD.
Answer: The steps include patient education, catheter placement, choosing an appropriate dialysis prescription, and monitoring for complications such as peritonitis.
Explanation: Practical knowledge of dialysis initiation is crucial for nephrologists and renal nurses.

39. Interpret the following urinalysis findings in a patient with suspected nephrotic syndrome: Protein 4+, RBCs 0-1/hpf, WBCs 2-3/hpf, No casts.
Answer: The findings are consistent with nephrotic syndrome, as indicated by significant proteinuria without hematuria or pyuria.
Explanation: Proper interpretation of urinalysis results is key in diagnosing and managing renal conditions.

40. Discuss the evidence supporting the use of ACE inhibitors in slowing the progression of CKD.
Answer: Multiple studies have shown that ACE inhibitors reduce proteinuria and slow CKD progression, particularly in patients with diabetes or proteinuria. This effect is due to the reduction of glomerular capillary pressure and antifibrotic effects.
Explanation: Understanding evidence-based practices ensures optimal patient outcomes in nephrology.

41. How would you explain the need for dialysis to a patient with newly diagnosed ESRD?
Answer: I would explain that dialysis is a treatment that performs the kidney's function of removing waste products and excess fluid from the blood when the kidneys are no longer able to do so. It is a life-saving therapy that can help

manage symptoms and improve quality of life.
Explanation: Clear and empathetic communication is essential in discussing treatment options with patients.

42. What are the differential diagnoses for a patient presenting with hematuria, proteinuria, and renal impairment?

Answer: Differential diagnoses include glomerulonephritis, lupus nephritis, IgA nephropathy, and membranous nephropathy.

Explanation: Identifying the correct diagnosis requires careful consideration of the clinical presentation and diagnostic tests.

43. In a patient with CKD and hyperkalemia, which of the following treatments should be prioritized?

Answer: Stabilizing the myocardium with calcium gluconate should be the first priority, followed by measures to reduce serum potassium levels.

Explanation: Immediate treatment to prevent arrhythmias is critical in managing hyperkalemia.

44. What are the risk factors for developing contrast-induced nephropathy?

Answer: Risk factors include pre-existing CKD, diabetes mellitus, dehydration, and the use of high doses of contrast media.

Explanation: Identifying and mitigating risk factors can help prevent this common iatrogenic complication.

45. Synthesize a management plan for a patient with acute glomerulonephritis presenting with hypertension, edema, and hematuria.

Answer: The management plan should include blood pressure control (preferably with an ACE inhibitor),

diuretics for edema, and possibly immunosuppressive therapy depending on the underlying cause. Monitoring renal function and adjusting treatment based on response is essential.
Explanation: A comprehensive approach is necessary for managing complex renal conditions.

46. Interpret the following lab results: Serum calcium 8.0 mg/dL, Serum phosphate 6.5 mg/dL, PTH 200 pg/mL in a patient with CKD.
Answer: These results suggest secondary hyperparathyroidism due to CKD, characterized by hypocalcemia, hyperphosphatemia, and elevated parathyroid hormone (PTH) levels.
Explanation: Managing mineral and bone disorders is a key aspect of CKD management.

47. A patient on hemodialysis develops hypotension during the session. What could be the cause and how would you address it?
Answer: Causes could include excessive fluid removal, autonomic dysfunction, or low cardiac output. Management includes reducing the ultrafiltration rate, administering fluids, and reassessing the dialysis prescription.
Explanation: Prompt identification and management of dialysis-related complications are crucial for patient safety.

48. A patient with CKD presents with worsening anemia despite erythropoiesis-stimulating agent (ESA) therapy. What should be the next step in management?
Answer: Evaluate for other causes of anemia, such as iron deficiency, inflammation, or blood loss. Check iron studies and consider IV iron supplementation if indicated.
Explanation: ESA resistance is often due to iron deficiency, and appropriate management can optimize patient

outcomes.

49. Evaluate the role of sodium bicarbonate in the treatment of metabolic acidosis in CKD.
Answer: Sodium bicarbonate is used to correct metabolic acidosis in CKD, which can slow disease progression and improve muscle function. However, it should be used cautiously in patients with volume overload or hypertension.
Explanation: The benefits and risks of treatment options must be carefully weighed in CKD management.

50. Integrate current guidelines into the management of a patient with diabetic nephropathy.
Answer: Current guidelines recommend strict blood pressure control (<130/80 mmHg), preferably with an ACE inhibitor or ARB, along with tight glycemic control and lifestyle modifications to manage diabetic nephropathy.
Explanation: Following evidence-based guidelines ensures standardized and effective care.

51. How would you adapt the management of a hypertensive patient with CKD who develops hyperkalemia on an ACE inhibitor?
Answer: Consider lowering the dose of the ACE inhibitor, adding a diuretic to promote potassium excretion, or switching to a different antihypertensive that does not increase potassium levels.
Explanation: Balancing blood pressure control with the risk of hyperkalemia requires careful medication management.

52. How does the concept of "nephron loss" contribute to the progression of chronic kidney disease?
Answer: Nephron loss leads to hyperfiltration in the

remaining nephrons, which increases glomerular pressure, promotes sclerosis, and accelerates the decline in renal function, perpetuating the cycle of CKD progression.
Explanation: Understanding the pathophysiological mechanisms of CKD progression is crucial for effective management.

53. A study shows a relative risk reduction of 30% for cardiovascular events in CKD patients treated with statins. Interpret this finding.
Answer: The relative risk reduction indicates that statin therapy reduces the risk of cardiovascular events by 30% in CKD patients compared to those not treated with statins. This supports the use of statins in this population to reduce cardiovascular risk.
Explanation: Interpreting statistical data helps in applying research findings to clinical practice.

54. Describe the pathogenesis of nephrotic syndrome.
Answer: Nephrotic syndrome is caused by increased glomerular permeability, leading to massive proteinuria, hypoalbuminemia, and subsequent edema. The loss of proteins such as albumin results in reduced oncotic pressure and fluid leakage into tissues.
Explanation: Understanding the underlying mechanisms of diseases is essential for diagnosis and treatment.

55. Compare the benefits and risks of kidney transplantation versus long-term dialysis in ESRD patients.
Answer: Kidney transplantation offers better quality of life and long-term survival compared to dialysis but carries risks such as surgical complications, rejection, and the need for lifelong immunosuppression. Dialysis is less invasive but associated with lower survival rates and a higher burden of treatment-related complications.

Explanation: Comparing treatment options is crucial for informed decision-making in ESRD.

56. How would you apply KDIGO guidelines in the management of a patient with CKD and albuminuria?
Answer: According to KDIGO guidelines, the patient should be treated with an ACE inhibitor or ARB to reduce proteinuria and slow CKD progression, along with blood pressure and glycemic control. Regular monitoring of renal function and albuminuria is recommended.
Explanation: Adhering to guidelines ensures that patients receive care based on the best available evidence.

57.: A 56-year-old man with a history of hypertension presents with swelling of the legs and foamy urine. Laboratory tests reveal a serum albumin level of 2.0 g/dL, proteinuria of 4.5 g/day, and hyperlipidemia.
What is the most likely diagnosis?
- A) Acute glomerulonephritis
- B) Nephrotic syndrome
- C) Chronic kidney disease
- D) Nephritic syndrome

Answer: B) Nephrotic syndrome

Explanation: The clinical presentation of significant proteinuria (>3.5 g/day), hypoalbuminemia, hyperlipidemia, and edema is characteristic of nephrotic syndrome. Nephrotic syndrome can result from conditions like minimal change disease, focal segmental glomerulosclerosis, and membranous nephropathy.

58: A 23-year-old woman presents with hematuria and mild hypertension. She recently had a sore throat. Urinalysis reveals dysmorphic red blood cells and red cell casts.
What is the most likely diagnosis?

- A) IgA nephropathy
- B) Post-streptococcal glomerulonephritis
- C) Lupus nephritis
- D) Goodpasture syndrome

Answer: B) Post-streptococcal glomerulonephritis

Explanation: Post-streptococcal glomerulonephritis typically occurs 1-3 weeks after a streptococcal infection, such as pharyngitis. The presence of hematuria, hypertension, and red cell casts in the urine are indicative of glomerular injury, which is consistent with this diagnosis.

59: A 45-year-old man with diabetes presents with a 5-year history of progressive proteinuria. His creatinine has recently increased from 1.1 mg/dL to 1.8 mg/dL. Urinalysis shows 3+ protein but no casts.
What is the most likely cause of his renal disease?
- A) Diabetic nephropathy
- B) Focal segmental glomerulosclerosis
- C) Membranous nephropathy
- D) Hypertensive nephrosclerosis

Answer: A) Diabetic nephropathy

Explanation: Diabetic nephropathy is the leading cause of chronic kidney disease in diabetic patients. It is characterized by progressive proteinuria, declining glomerular filtration rate (GFR), and eventual kidney failure. The absence of casts suggests that the proteinuria is not due to glomerulonephritis but rather a condition like diabetic nephropathy.

60: A 60-year-old male with a history of chronic kidney disease presents with severe hyperkalemia (K+ = 6.8 mmol/L).
Which of the following should be administered first?

- A) Insulin and glucose
- B) Calcium gluconate
- C) Sodium bicarbonate
- D) Kayexalate

Answer: B) Calcium gluconate

Explanation: In the setting of severe hyperkalemia, calcium gluconate should be administered first to stabilize the cardiac membrane and prevent arrhythmias. Following this, insulin and glucose, sodium bicarbonate, and other therapies can be used to lower potassium levels.

61: A 35-year-old woman with systemic lupus erythematosus (SLE) presents with nephrotic range proteinuria, hematuria, and renal insufficiency.

What is the most likely diagnosis?
- A) Lupus nephritis
- B) Minimal change disease
- C) Membranous nephropathy
- D) IgA nephropathy

Answer: A) Lupus nephritis

Explanation: Lupus nephritis is a common and serious complication of SLE. It typically presents with proteinuria, hematuria, and progressive renal dysfunction. Renal biopsy is often necessary to classify the severity and guide treatment.

62: A 52-year-old man presents with fatigue and pruritus. Laboratory results reveal elevated blood urea nitrogen (BUN) and creatinine, hyperphosphatemia, hypocalcemia, and anemia.

What is the most likely diagnosis?
- A) Acute kidney injury
- B) Chronic kidney disease

- C) Primary hyperparathyroidism
- D) Nephrotic syndrome

Answer: B) Chronic kidney disease

Explanation: Chronic kidney disease (CKD) often presents with symptoms related to uremia, such as fatigue and pruritus. Laboratory findings typically include elevated BUN and creatinine, hyperphosphatemia, hypocalcemia, and anemia due to reduced erythropoietin production.

63: A 70-year-old man presents with flank pain, hematuria, and a palpable mass in the abdomen.

What is the most likely diagnosis?
- A) Renal cell carcinoma
- B) Polycystic kidney disease
- C) Pyelonephritis
- D) Renal vein thrombosis

Answer: A) Renal cell carcinoma

Explanation: The classic triad of renal cell carcinoma includes flank pain, hematuria, and a palpable abdominal mass. Renal cell carcinoma is the most common type of kidney cancer in adults.

64: A 40-year-old woman with no significant medical history presents with sudden onset of severe right-sided flank pain radiating to the groin. Urinalysis shows microscopic hematuria.

What is the most likely diagnosis?
- A) Renal stone
- B) Pyelonephritis
- C) Hydronephrosis
- D) Renal artery stenosis

Answer: A) Renal stone

Explanation: The sudden onset of severe flank pain radiating to the groin, along with hematuria, is typical of nephrolithiasis (renal stone). The pain results from the stone passing through the ureter, causing obstruction and spasm.

65: A 68-year-old woman with a history of diabetes and hypertension presents with generalized edema and difficulty breathing. Urinalysis reveals 4+ proteinuria and fatty casts. Serum creatinine is 3.0 mg/dL.

What is the most appropriate next step in management?
- A) ACE inhibitor therapy
- B) Renal biopsy
- C) Start dialysis
- D) Fluid restriction

Answer: B) Renal biopsy

Explanation: This patient's clinical presentation is consistent with nephrotic syndrome. A renal biopsy is necessary to determine the underlying cause, especially given the presence of significant proteinuria, renal dysfunction, and edema.

66: A 54-year-old man presents with fatigue, anorexia, and difficulty concentrating. His laboratory results reveal a GFR of 15 mL/min/1.73 m².

What stage of chronic kidney disease (CKD) is this patient in?
- A) Stage 2
- B) Stage 3
- C) Stage 4
- D) Stage 5

Answer: D) Stage 5

Explanation: Chronic kidney disease is classified into five stages based on GFR. Stage 5 CKD, also known as end-stage renal disease (ESRD), is characterized by a GFR of less than 15 mL/min/1.73 m², at which point dialysis or kidney transplantation may be required.

67: A 25-year-old man presents with hemoptysis, hematuria, and rapidly progressive renal failure.

What is the most likely diagnosis?
- A) Goodpasture syndrome
- B) Wegener's granulomatosis
- C) IgA nephropathy
- D) Lupus nephritis

Answer: A) Goodpasture syndrome

Explanation: Goodpasture syndrome is characterized by the presence of anti-glomerular basement membrane antibodies leading to rapidly progressive glomerulonephritis and pulmonary hemorrhage. Hemoptysis and hematuria are key clinical features.

68: A 65-year-old man with a history of hypertension presents with a blood pressure of 180/110 mmHg, and serum potassium of 2.8 mmol/L. He is on hydrochlorothiazide.

What is the most likely cause of his hypokalemia?
- A) Hyperaldosteronism
- B) Renal artery stenosis
- C) Hypomagnesemia
- D) Renal tubular acidosis

Answer: A) Hyperaldosteronism

Explanation: Hyperaldosteronism, often due to an adrenal adenoma (Conn's syndrome), can cause hypertension and hypokalemia. The excess aldosterone increases sodium reabsorption at the expense of potassium, leading to hypokalemia.

69: A 28-year-old woman presents with recurrent episodes of hematuria, often associated with upper respiratory infections.

What is the most likely diagnosis?
- A) IgA nephropathy
- B) Post-streptococcal glomerulonephritis
- C) Lupus nephritis
- D) Membranous nephropathy

Answer: A) IgA nephropathy

Explanation: IgA nephropathy (Berger's disease) often presents with recurrent episodes of hematuria, particularly following upper respiratory infections. It is the most common cause of glomerulonephritis worldwide.

70: A 45-year-old man with a history of multiple myeloma presents with renal failure.
What is the most likely cause of his renal dysfunction?
- A) Light chain nephropathy (myeloma kidney)
- B) Amyloidosis
- C) Hypercalcemia
- D) Urinary tract infection

Answer: A) Light chain nephropathy (myeloma kidney)

Explanation: In multiple myeloma, excess light chains are produced and filtered by the kidneys, leading to cast formation and tubular obstruction, known as myeloma kidney. This is a common cause of renal failure in patients with multiple myeloma.

71: A 35-year-old woman presents with new-onset hypertension. Her laboratory tests reveal hypokalemia and metabolic alkalosis.
What is the most likely cause of her condition?
- A) Conn's syndrome (primary hyperaldosteronism)
- B) Cushing's syndrome
- C) Renal artery stenosis

- D) Pheochromocytoma

Answer: A) Conn's syndrome (primary hyperaldosteronism)

Explanation: Conn's syndrome is characterized by excessive aldosterone production, leading to sodium retention, hypertension, hypokalemia, and metabolic alkalosis. It is a common cause of secondary hypertension.

72: A 30-year-old man with a history of polycystic kidney disease presents with sudden onset severe headache and collapse.

What is the most likely diagnosis?
- A) Subarachnoid hemorrhage
- B) Hypertensive encephalopathy
- C) Intracranial hemorrhage
- D) Ischemic stroke

Answer: A) Subarachnoid hemorrhage

Explanation: Patients with polycystic kidney disease (PKD) are at increased risk for intracranial aneurysms and subarachnoid hemorrhage. The sudden onset of severe headache ("thunderclap headache") and collapse is characteristic of a subarachnoid hemorrhage.

73: A 65-year-old man with a history of benign prostatic hyperplasia (BPH) presents with anuria and lower abdominal discomfort.

What is the most likely cause of his anuria?
- A) Acute tubular necrosis
- B) Obstructive uropathy
- C) Renal artery stenosis
- D) Dehydration

Answer: B) Obstructive uropathy

Explanation: In patients with BPH, obstruction of the urinary tract can lead to obstructive uropathy, characterized by anuria or oliguria and bladder distension. Relief of the obstruction is necessary to restore renal function.

74: A 58-year-old man with long-standing diabetes presents with swelling of the legs, proteinuria, and a creatinine of 2.2 mg/dL.

What is the most likely renal lesion seen on biopsy?

- A) Nodular glomerulosclerosis (Kimmelstiel-Wilson lesion)
- B) Membranous nephropathy
- C) Focal segmental glomerulosclerosis
- D) Minimal change disease

Answer: A) Nodular glomerulosclerosis (Kimmelstiel-Wilson lesion)

Explanation: Nodular glomerulosclerosis, also known as Kimmelstiel-Wilson lesion, is a hallmark of diabetic nephropathy. It is characterized by nodular deposits in the glomeruli and is associated with significant proteinuria.

75: A 24-year-old woman presents with acute kidney injury, microangiopathic hemolytic anemia, and thrombocytopenia.

What is the most likely diagnosis?

- A) Hemolytic uremic syndrome (HUS)
- B) Thrombotic thrombocytopenic purpura (TTP)
- C) Systemic lupus erythematosus
- D) Disseminated intravascular coagulation (DIC)

Answer: A) Hemolytic uremic syndrome (HUS)

Explanation: Hemolytic uremic syndrome (HUS) is characterized by the triad of acute kidney injury, microangiopathic hemolytic anemia, and thrombocytopenia. It is often associated with infections, particularly Shiga toxin-producing Escherichia coli.

76: A 50-year-old man with a history of chronic hypertension presents with elevated creatinine and small, shrunken kidneys on ultrasound.

What is the most likely diagnosis?
- A) Hypertensive nephrosclerosis
- B) Chronic pyelonephritis
- C) Diabetic nephropathy
- D) Polycystic kidney disease

Answer: A) Hypertensive nephrosclerosis

Explanation: Hypertensive nephrosclerosis is a common cause of chronic kidney disease, particularly in patients with long-standing hypertension. The kidneys are typically small and shrunken due to chronic ischemic injury.

77: A 45-year-old man presents with flank pain and a history of recurrent kidney stones. He is found to have hypercalcemia.

What is the most likely underlying condition?
- A) Hyperparathyroidism
- B) Sarcoidosis
- C) Multiple myeloma
- D) Vitamin D intoxication

Answer: A) Hyperparathyroidism

Explanation: Primary hyperparathyroidism is a common cause of hypercalcemia and is often associated with kidney stones due to hypercalciuria. The presence of flank pain and recurrent stones in the setting of hypercalcemia is suggestive of this diagnosis.

78: A 30-year-old woman with systemic lupus erythematosus presents with hematuria, proteinuria, and a decline in renal function.

Which test is most helpful in assessing the extent of renal involvement?

- A) Renal biopsy
- B) Serum complement levels
- C) Anti-dsDNA antibodies
- D) Urinalysis

Answer: A) Renal biopsy

Explanation: Renal biopsy is the gold standard for assessing the extent and type of renal involvement in lupus nephritis. It helps guide treatment by identifying the specific class of lupus nephritis.

79: A 60-year-old man with a history of heart failure presents with hyperkalemia. His current medications include lisinopril, spironolactone, furosemide, and digoxin.

Which medication is most likely contributing to his hyperkalemia?

- A) Lisinopril
- B) Furosemide
- C) Digoxin
- D) Spironolactone

Answer: D) Spironolactone

Explanation: Spironolactone, an aldosterone antagonist, can cause hyperkalemia, especially in patients with reduced renal function or those taking other medications that also increase potassium levels, such as ACE inhibitors like lisinopril.

80: A 70-year-old woman presents with confusion, lethargy, and muscle weakness. Her laboratory results show a sodium level of 115 mmol/L.

What is the most appropriate initial treatment?

- A) Hypertonic saline
- B) Fluid restriction
- C) Demeclocycline
- D) Normal saline

Answer: A) Hypertonic saline

Explanation: Severe hyponatremia (Na+ <120 mmol/L) with symptoms such as confusion and lethargy should be treated with hypertonic saline to rapidly increase serum sodium levels and prevent complications like cerebral edema.

81: A 55-year-old man presents with oliguria, elevated creatinine, and a history of non-steroidal anti-inflammatory drug (NSAID) use.

What is the most likely diagnosis?

- A) Acute interstitial nephritis
- B) Acute tubular necrosis
- C) Chronic glomerulonephritis
- D) Post-renal obstruction

Answer: A) Acute interstitial nephritis

Explanation: Acute interstitial nephritis is commonly associated with NSAID use and presents with oliguria, elevated creatinine, and sometimes allergic-type symptoms such as rash and eosinophilia. Discontinuing the offending drug is essential.

82: A 40-year-old woman presents with recurrent kidney stones composed of calcium oxalate.

Which dietary modification is most appropriate to reduce her risk of future stones?

- A) Increase dietary calcium
- B) Decrease dietary oxalate
- C) Increase protein intake

- D) Decrease dietary calcium

Answer: B) Decrease dietary oxalate

Explanation: Reducing dietary oxalate is an important strategy in preventing calcium oxalate stones. Foods high in oxalate, such as spinach, nuts, and chocolate, should be limited.

83: A 22-year-old man presents with a history of recurrent hematuria and a hearing deficit. His father had a similar condition and developed kidney failure in his 40s.

What is the most likely diagnosis?

- A) Alport syndrome
- B) IgA nephropathy
- C) Thin basement membrane disease
- D) Polycystic kidney disease

Answer: A) Alport syndrome

Explanation: Alport syndrome is a genetic disorder characterized by progressive renal disease, hearing loss, and eye abnormalities. The family history of similar symptoms and kidney failure is consistent with this diagnosis.

84: A 50-year-old woman with a history of type 2 diabetes presents with proteinuria, hematuria, and a normal-sized kidney on ultrasound.

Which of the following is the most appropriate initial treatment to slow the progression of her renal disease?

- A) High-dose corticosteroids
- B) Angiotensin-converting enzyme (ACE) inhibitor
- C) Calcium channel blocker
- D) Diuretic

Answer: B) Angiotensin-converting enzyme (ACE) inhibitor

Explanation: In patients with diabetic nephropathy, ACE inhibitors are effective in reducing proteinuria and slowing the progression of renal disease by decreasing intraglomerular pressure and providing renal protection.

85: A 45-year-old man presents with low back pain, and his lab tests reveal a serum calcium of 12.5 mg/dL and elevated parathyroid hormone (PTH) levels.

What is the most likely cause of his hypercalcemia?
- A) Primary hyperparathyroidism
- B) Vitamin D toxicity
- C) Multiple myeloma
- D) Secondary hyperparathyroidism

Answer: A) Primary hyperparathyroidism

Explanation: Primary hyperparathyroidism is characterized by elevated calcium levels and elevated PTH. It is often associated with hypercalcemia and can cause symptoms like bone pain and kidney stones.

86: A 60-year-old man presents with a history of hypertension and new-onset proteinuria. A kidney biopsy reveals segmental glomerular scarring.

What is the most likely diagnosis?
- A) Focal segmental glomerulosclerosis (FSGS)
- B) Membranous nephropathy
- C) Minimal change disease
- D) Diabetic nephropathy

Answer: A) Focal segmental glomerulosclerosis (FSGS)

Explanation: Focal segmental glomerulosclerosis is characterized by segmental scarring of glomeruli and can present with nephrotic syndrome and hypertension. It is a common cause of proteinuria and renal impairment.

87: A 25-year-old man with a history of recent viral illness presents with hematuria and flank pain. Urinalysis shows red blood cell casts.

What is the most likely diagnosis?
- A) Acute glomerulonephritis
- B) Nephrolithiasis
- C) Pyelonephritis
- D) Renal cell carcinoma

Answer: A) Acute glomerulonephritis

Explanation: Red blood cell casts are indicative of glomerular inflammation. Acute glomerulonephritis often follows a viral infection and is characterized by hematuria, red cell casts, and sometimes proteinuria.

88: A 55-year-old woman with a history of rheumatoid arthritis presents with renal failure, anemia, and a "bubbly" appearance on renal ultrasound.

What is the most likely diagnosis?
- A) Amyloidosis
- B) Chronic pyelonephritis
- C) Renal cell carcinoma
- D) Polycystic kidney disease

Answer: A) Amyloidosis

Explanation: Amyloidosis can present with renal involvement characterized by nephrotic syndrome and renal failure. The "bubbly" appearance on ultrasound refers to renal echogenicity changes associated with amyloid deposition.

89: A 30-year-old man with a history of recurrent urinary tract infections presents with fever, flank pain, and nausea. A renal ultrasound shows an enlarged kidney with multiple abscesses.

What is the most appropriate initial treatment?
- A) Intravenous antibiotics
- B) Oral antibiotics
- C) Nephrectomy
- D) Urinary tract drainage

Answer: A) Intravenous antibiotics

Explanation: For a patient with pyelonephritis complicated by abscess formation, intravenous antibiotics are required to address severe infection and ensure adequate tissue penetration.

90: A 45-year-old woman presents with fatigue, pruritus, and evidence of metabolic bone disease. Her laboratory tests reveal elevated phosphate and low calcium.

What is the most likely diagnosis?
- A) Chronic kidney disease
- B) Hyperparathyroidism
- C) Osteomalacia
- D) Hypervitaminosis D

Answer: A) Chronic kidney disease

Explanation: In chronic kidney disease, the kidneys fail to excrete phosphate properly, leading to secondary hyperparathyroidism and resultant low serum calcium and elevated phosphate levels. This causes bone metabolism issues.

91: A 40-year-old man with a history of diabetes presents with worsening renal function and evidence of an abnormality on renal imaging.

What is the most likely finding on renal imaging if he has diabetic nephropathy?
- A) Normal-sized kidneys
- B) Enlarged kidneys

- C) Cysts
- D) Renal artery stenosis

Answer: A) Normal-sized kidneys

Explanation: Diabetic nephropathy often presents with normal or slightly reduced kidney size on imaging, unlike polycystic kidney disease which shows enlarged kidneys or renal artery stenosis that might show narrowed renal arteries.

92: A 50-year-old man presents with hypertension, hyperkalemia, and a history of heart failure. He is on a potassium-sparing diuretic.

What is the most likely cause of his hyperkalemia?
- A) Potassium-sparing diuretic
- B) Renal artery stenosis
- C) Excessive potassium intake
- D) Acute kidney injury

Answer: A) Potassium-sparing diuretic

Explanation: Potassium-sparing diuretics, such as spironolactone, can lead to hyperkalemia by reducing potassium excretion. This is especially problematic in patients with pre-existing renal impairment or those taking other potassium-sparing medications.

93: A 35-year-old man with a history of recurrent kidney stones is found to have elevated uric acid levels.

What dietary modification should he consider to reduce his stone risk?
- A) Increase intake of animal protein
- B) Decrease intake of purine-rich foods
- C) Increase intake of calcium

- D) Decrease intake of fluids

Answer: B) Decrease intake of purine-rich foods

Explanation: Elevated uric acid levels can lead to uric acid stones. Reducing intake of purine-rich foods (e.g., red meat, seafood) helps decrease uric acid levels and prevent stone formation.

94: A 28-year-old woman with a history of systemic lupus erythematosus presents with worsening renal function and new-onset proteinuria.

Which autoantibody test is most likely to be positive in this patient?

- A) Anti-dsDNA antibodies
- B) Anti-Smith antibodies
- C) Anti-SSA/Ro antibodies
- D) Anti-SSB/La antibodies

Answer: A) Anti-dsDNA antibodies

Explanation: Anti-dsDNA antibodies are commonly associated with lupus nephritis and can be elevated in patients with worsening renal function due to SLE.

95: A 40-year-old man with a history of gout presents with acute onset of flank pain and hematuria.

What is the most likely diagnosis?

- A) Uric acid nephrolithiasis
- B) Acute pyelonephritis
- C) Calcium oxalate nephrolithiasis
- D) Acute glomerulonephritis

Answer: A) Uric acid nephrolithiasis

Explanation: Gout is associated with elevated uric acid levels, which can lead to the formation of uric acid stones in the kidneys. These stones can cause acute pain and hematuria.

96: A 65-year-old man with a history of hypertension presents with edema and a urine dipstick showing 2+ protein. His renal function tests are normal.

What is the most likely cause of his proteinuria?
- A) Orthostatic proteinuria
- B) Nephrotic syndrome
- C) Glomerulonephritis
- D) Diabetes mellitus

Answer: A) Orthostatic proteinuria

Explanation: Orthostatic proteinuria is common in younger individuals and is characterized by the presence of protein in the urine that occurs only when the patient is upright. In older patients, this is less common but still a possibility in the absence of other symptoms or renal function abnormalities.

97: A 50-year-old woman presents with hypertension, low-grade fever, and flank pain. Her renal ultrasound shows multiple small, well-defined cysts in both kidneys.

What is the most appropriate next step in management?
- A) Reassurance and regular follow-up
- B) Initiate antihypertensive therapy
- C) Start antibiotics
- D) Renal biopsy

Answer: A) Reassurance and regular follow-up

Explanation: The presence of multiple small, well-defined cysts on ultrasound is typical of simple renal cysts. These usually require no specific treatment, just periodic monitoring to ensure they do not change significantly.

98: A 30-year-old man presents with a history of recurrent urinary tract infections and a solitary functioning kidney.

What is the most important preventive measure to reduce the risk of future infections?
- A) Regular urinalysis
- B) Prophylactic antibiotics
- C) Increase fluid intake
- D) Avoidance of NSAIDs

Answer: C) Increase fluid intake

Explanation: Increasing fluid intake helps flush out bacteria from the urinary tract, reducing the risk of recurrent infections, especially in patients with a solitary functioning kidney.

99: A 70-year-old man with a history of benign prostatic hyperplasia presents with acute renal failure and a distended bladder.

What is the most likely cause of his acute renal failure?
- A) Post-renal obstruction
- B) Acute tubular necrosis
- C) Pre-renal azotemia
- D) Acute glomerulonephritis

Answer: A) Post-renal obstruction

Explanation: In patients with BPH, acute urinary retention can lead to post-renal obstruction and subsequent acute renal failure. Relief of the obstruction is necessary for renal function recovery.

100: A 40-year-old man with a history of chronic kidney disease presents with fatigue, shortness of breath, and an elevated serum creatinine level. He also has a low hemoglobin level.

What is the most likely cause of his anemia?
- A) Anemia of chronic disease
- B) Iron deficiency anemia
- C) Hemolytic anemia

- D) Vitamin B12 deficiency

Answer: A) Anemia of chronic disease

Explanation: Anemia in chronic kidney disease is often due to decreased erythropoietin production by the kidneys. It is a common form of anemia in patients with chronic renal impairment.

101: A 50-year-old woman presents with an elevated serum creatinine and a history of frequent headaches. She has been on a new medication for hypertension.

What is the most likely cause of her renal impairment?
- A) Drug-induced renal injury
- B) Chronic glomerulonephritis
- C) Renal artery stenosis
- D) Diabetic nephropathy

Answer: A) Drug-induced renal injury

Explanation: Certain antihypertensive drugs, particularly NSAIDs and ACE inhibitors, can cause renal impairment. If the patient recently started a new medication, it is important to consider drug-induced renal injury as a potential cause.

102: A 45-year-old man presents with new-onset hypertension and renal dysfunction. His laboratory tests show elevated serum creatinine and a urine albumin-to-creatinine ratio of 300 mg/g.

What is the most likely diagnosis?
- A) Chronic kidney disease
- B) Diabetic nephropathy
- C) Hypertensive nephrosclerosis
- D) Acute glomerulonephritis

Answer: C) Hypertensive nephrosclerosis

Explanation: Elevated urine albumin-to-creatinine ratio and renal dysfunction in the context of long-standing hypertension suggest hypertensive nephrosclerosis. This condition is a result of chronic high blood pressure causing progressive renal damage.

103: A 65-year-old woman presents with new-onset edema and a serum creatinine level of 1.8 mg/dL. She has a history of rheumatoid arthritis and is on methotrexate.

What is the most appropriate next step in management?
- A) Discontinue methotrexate
- B) Initiate corticosteroids
- C) Start dialysis
- D) Perform a renal biopsy

Answer: A) Discontinue methotrexate

Explanation: Methotrexate can cause renal impairment, especially in patients with pre-existing kidney issues. Discontinuing the offending drug is a crucial step in managing drug-induced renal dysfunction.

CHAPTER 15: REFERENCES

- Brenner BM, Rector FC. *Brenner & Rector's The Kidney*. 10th ed. Philadelphia, PA: Elsevier; 2015.
- Johnson RJ, Feehally J. *Comprehensive Clinical Nephrology*. 5th ed. St. Louis, MO: Elsevier; 2014.
- KDIGO Clinical Practice Guidelines for Glomerulonephritis. Kidney Int Suppl. 2012;2(2):139-274.
- Levey AS, Coresh J, Balk E, et al. National Kidney Foundation Practice Guidelines for Chronic Kidney Disease: Evaluation, Classification, and Stratification. Ann Intern Med. 2003;139(2):137-147.
- Taal MW, Chertow GM, Marsden PA, Skorecki K, Yu ASL, Brenner BM. *Brenner and Rector's The Kidney*. 9th ed. Saunders; 2011.

ABOUT THE AUTHOR

Dr Essam Abdelhakim

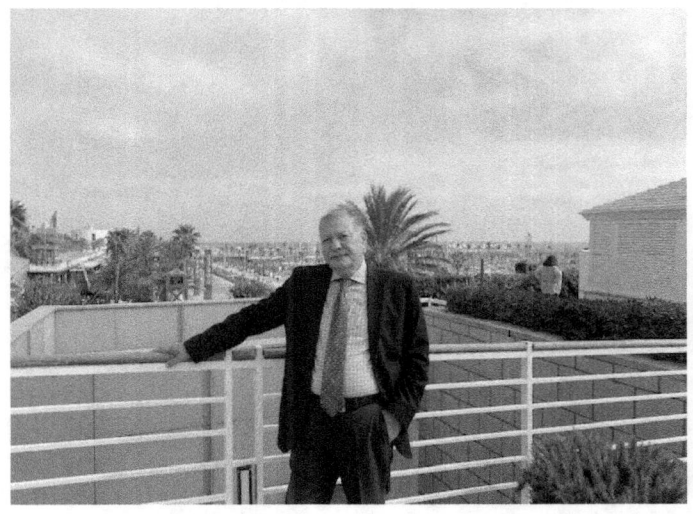

Senior Consultant and Expert in Medical Education